LONG BRANCH ELEMENTARY
MEDIA CENTER
33 N FILLMORE STREET
ARLINGTON, VA 22201

FOOD

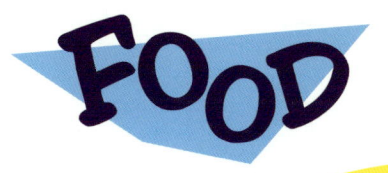

Dairy Products

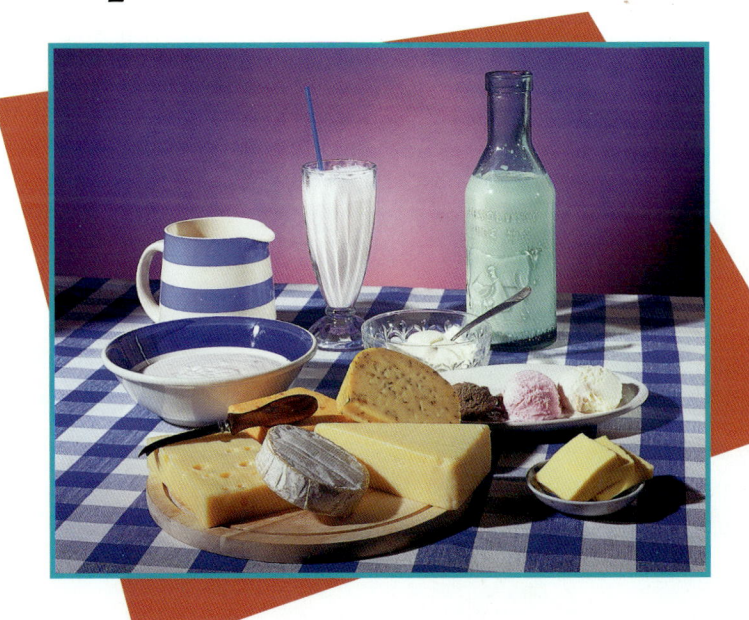

Ann Thomas

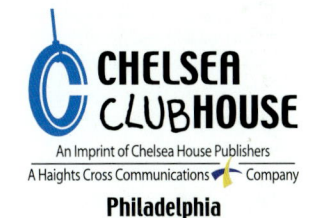

CHELSEA CLUBHOUSE
An Imprint of Chelsea House Publishers
A Haights Cross Communications Company

Philadelphia

This edition first published in 2003 in the United States of America by Chelsea Clubhouse, a division of Chelsea House Publishers and a subsidiary of Haights Cross Communications.

All rights reserved. No part of this publication may be reproduced or transmitted in any form or by any means without the written permission of the publisher.

Chelsea Clubhouse
1974 Sproul Road, Suite 400
Broomall, PA 19008-0914

The Chelsea House world wide web address is www.chelseahouse.com

Library of Congress Cataloging-in-Publication Data

Thomas, Ann, 1953-
   Dairy products / by Ann Thomas.
   p. cm. — (Food)

Includes index.
Summary: A simple introduction to such foods as milk, cheese, and yogurt that are part of the dairy products group of the USDA Food Guide Pyramid.

ISBN 0-7910-6980-X
1. Nutrition—Juvenile literature. 2. Dairy products—Juvenile literature. [1. Dairy products.] I. Title. II. Food (Philadelphia, Pa.)
TX355 .T4513 2003
613.2—dc21

                                                                                                   2002000025

First published in 1998 by
MACMILLAN EDUCATION AUSTRALIA PTY LTD
627 Chapel Street, South Yarra, Australia, 3141

Copyright © Ann Thomas 1998
Copyright in photographs © individual photographers as credited

Text design by Polar Design
Cover design by Linda Forss
Illustrations © Anthony Pike

Printed in China

Acknowledgements
Special thanks to Tom in the laboratories at National Dairies, Adelaide.

Cover: Great Southern Stock

Australian Dairy Corporation, p. 20; Australian Picture Library, pp. 8, 9, 22 ©ZEFA/Zentrale Photo, 19 ©Didier Givois, 25 ©Henryk T. Kaiser, 27 ©Guy Marche; Coo-ee Picture Library, p. 10; Corbis, p. 24; Ferrero-Labat/Auscape, 5; Getty Images, pp. 14, 18, 30; Great Southern Stock, pp. 11, 23, 26, 29, 28; HORIZON Photo Library, p. 16; MEA Photo, p. 15; The Photo Library-Sydney, p. 6 ©Jenny Mills, 12 ©Val Forman Photography, 13 ©Walter Glover, 14 ©Phillip Weir, 17 ©Nino Marshall, 21 ©CC Studio/SPL; U.S. Department of Agriculture (USDA), p. 7.

While every care has been taken to trace and acknowledge copyright, the publisher tenders their apologies for any accidental infringement where copyright has proved untraceable.

Contents

4   Why Do We Need Food?
6   What Do We Need to Eat?
8   Dairy Products
10 Where Milk Comes From
12 Processing Milk
14 Reduced Fat Milk
16 From the Farm to the Factory
18 Yogurt
19 Cheese
20 Butter
22 Drinking and Cooking with Milk
24 Eating and Cooking with Cheese
26 Cooking with Cream
28 Vegans
30 The Dairy Group
31 Glossary
32 Index

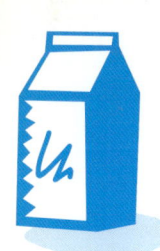

Why Do We Need Food?

We need food to keep us healthy. All living things need food and water to survive.

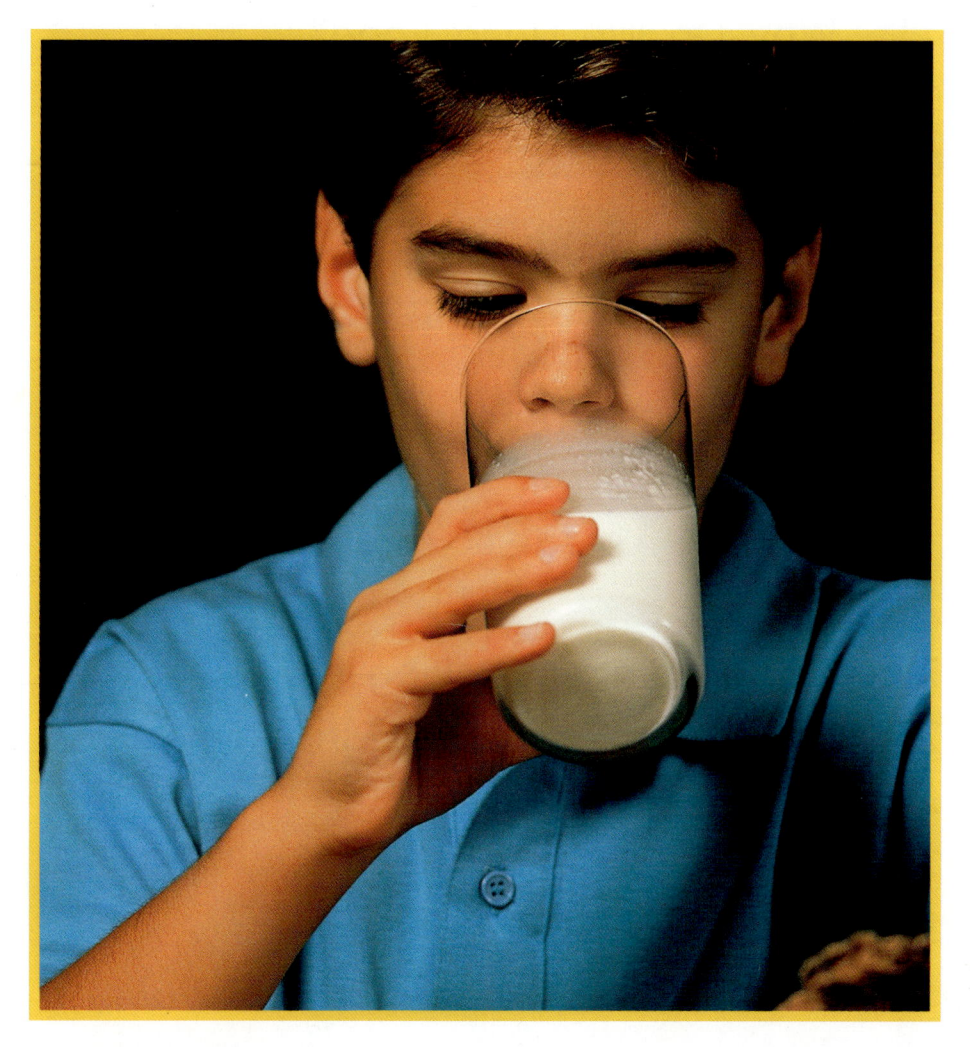

Milk and foods made from milk are called dairy products.

Giraffes eat tree leaves.

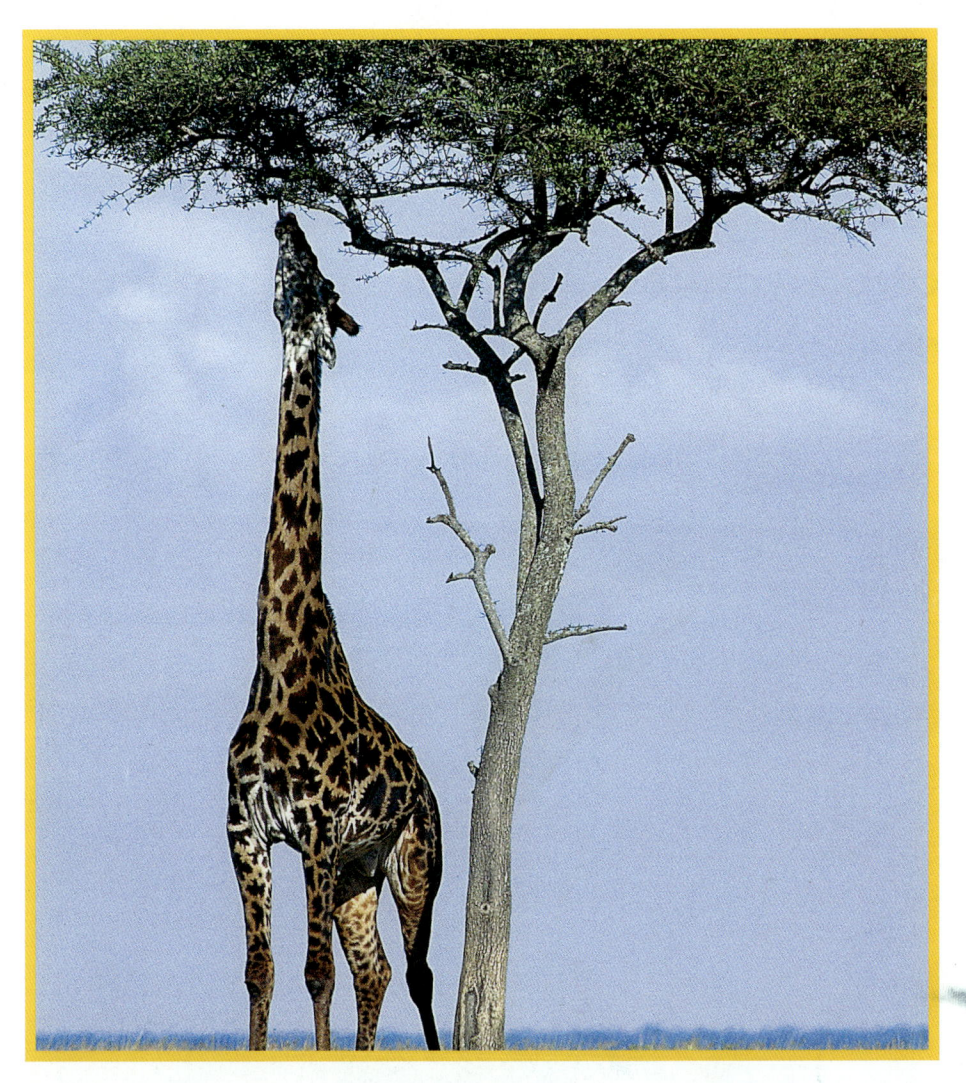

There are many kinds of food to eat. People, animals, and plants need different types of food.

5

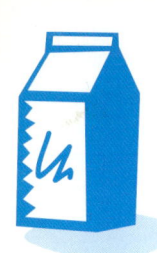

What Do We Need to Eat?

Foods can be put into groups. Some groups give us **vitamins** or **minerals**. Some groups give us **proteins** or **carbohydrates**. We need these **nutrients** to keep us healthy.

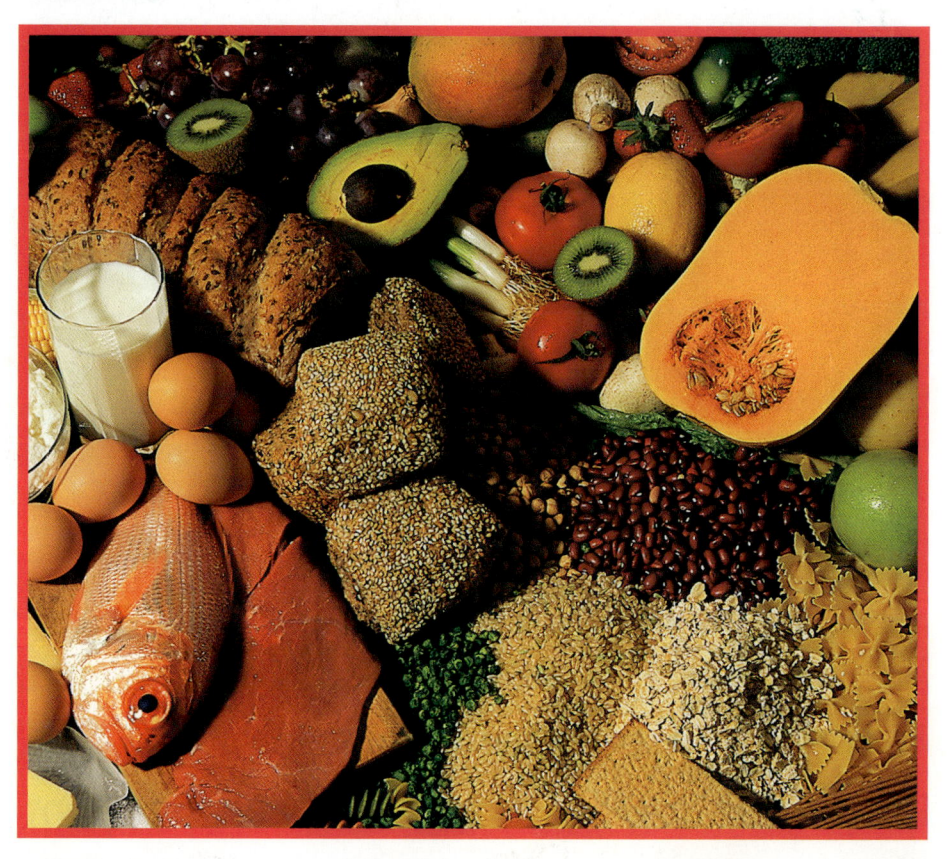

We need to eat a variety of foods.

Fats, Oils, and Sweets
use sparingly

Dairy Group
2–3 servings

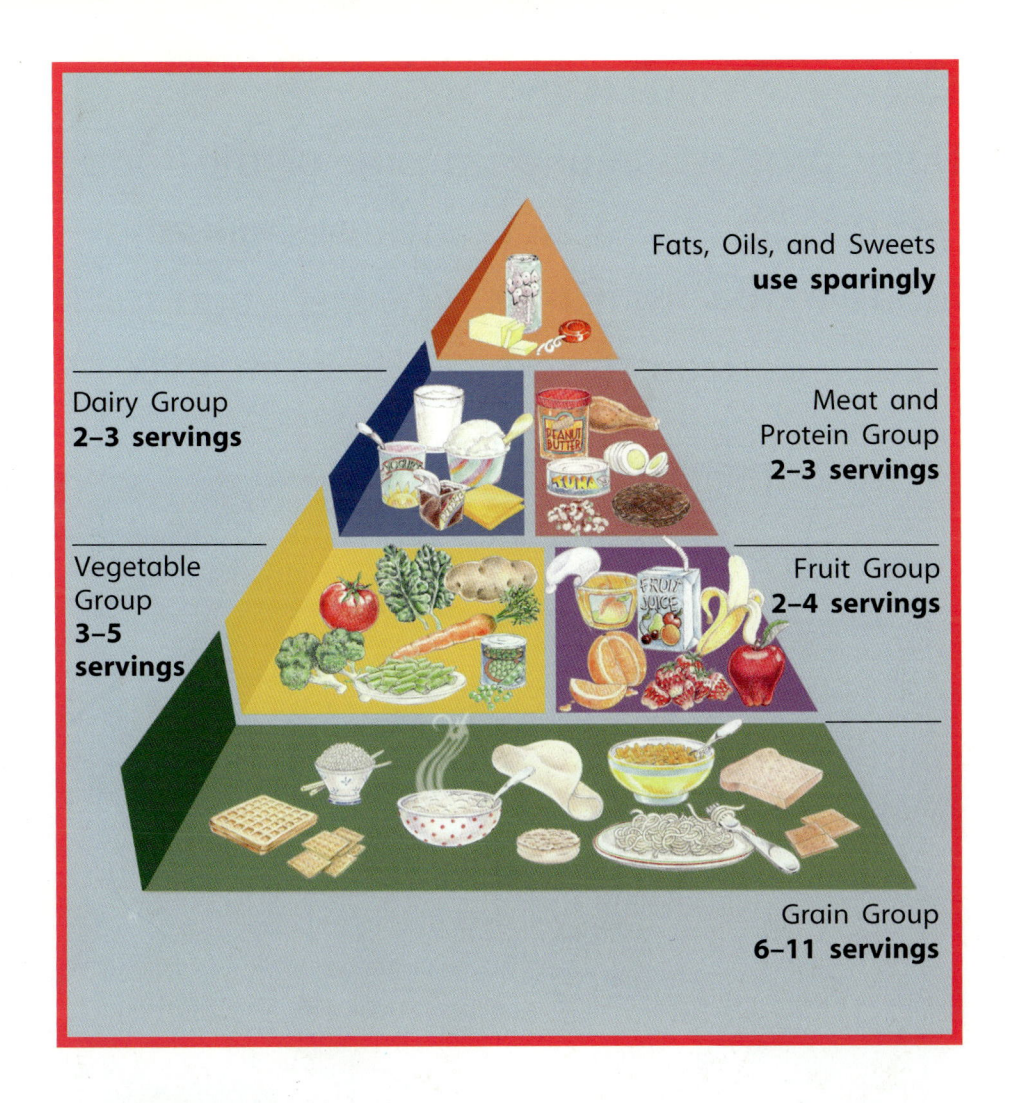

Meat and Protein Group
2–3 servings

Vegetable Group
3–5 servings

Fruit Group
2–4 servings

Grain Group
6–11 servings

The food guide pyramid shows us the food groups. We should eat the least from groups at the top. We should eat the most from groups at the bottom.

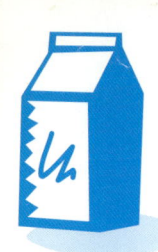

Dairy Products

Dairy products make up one of the food groups. Dairy products include milk and foods made from milk. Cheese, yogurt, cream, and butter are made from milk.

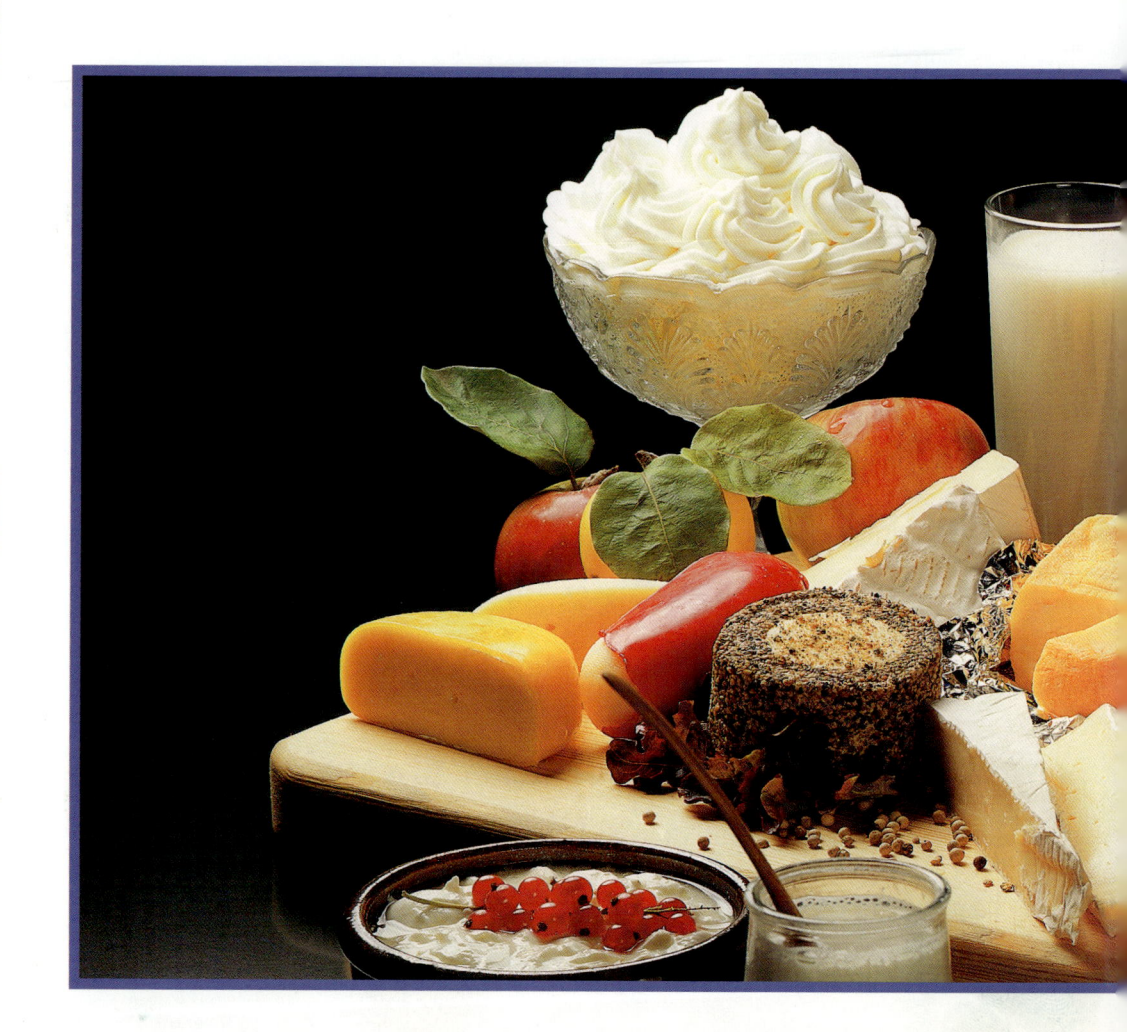

Most dairy foods contain proteins and vitamins. They also have minerals such as calcium. Calcium helps to keep our bones strong.

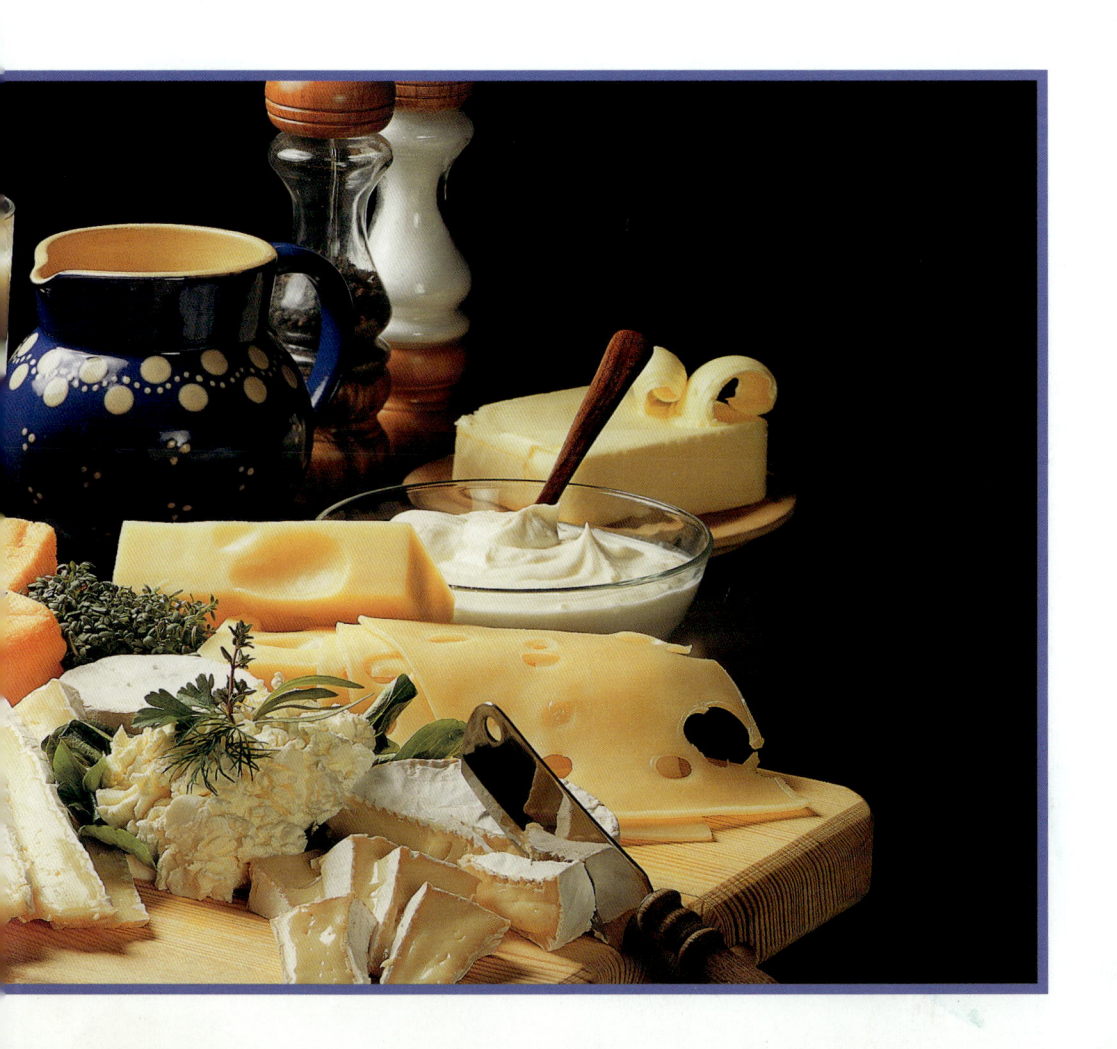

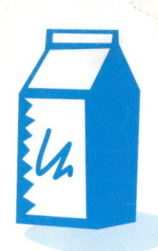

Where Milk Comes From

Most people drink milk that comes from dairy cows. Most dairy foods are made out of cow milk.

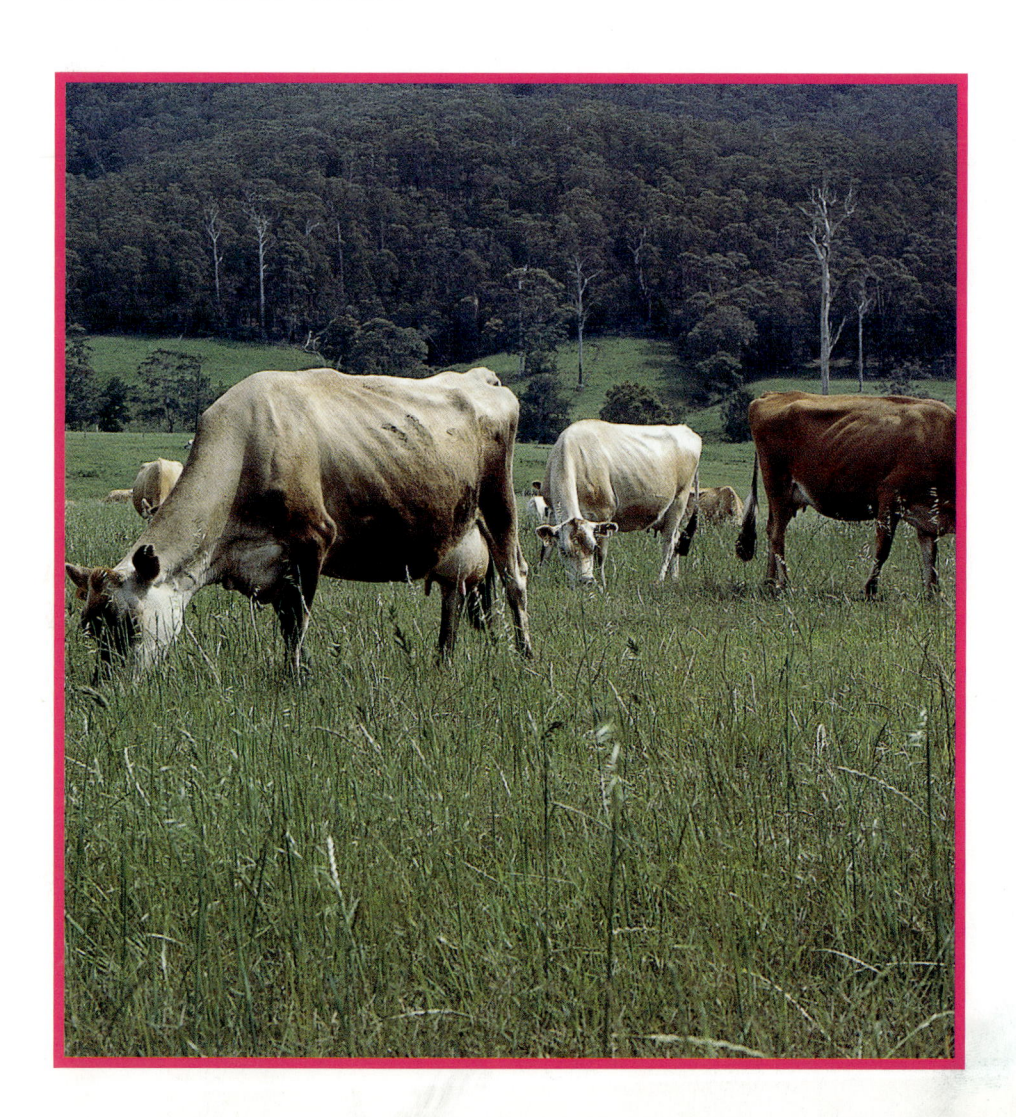

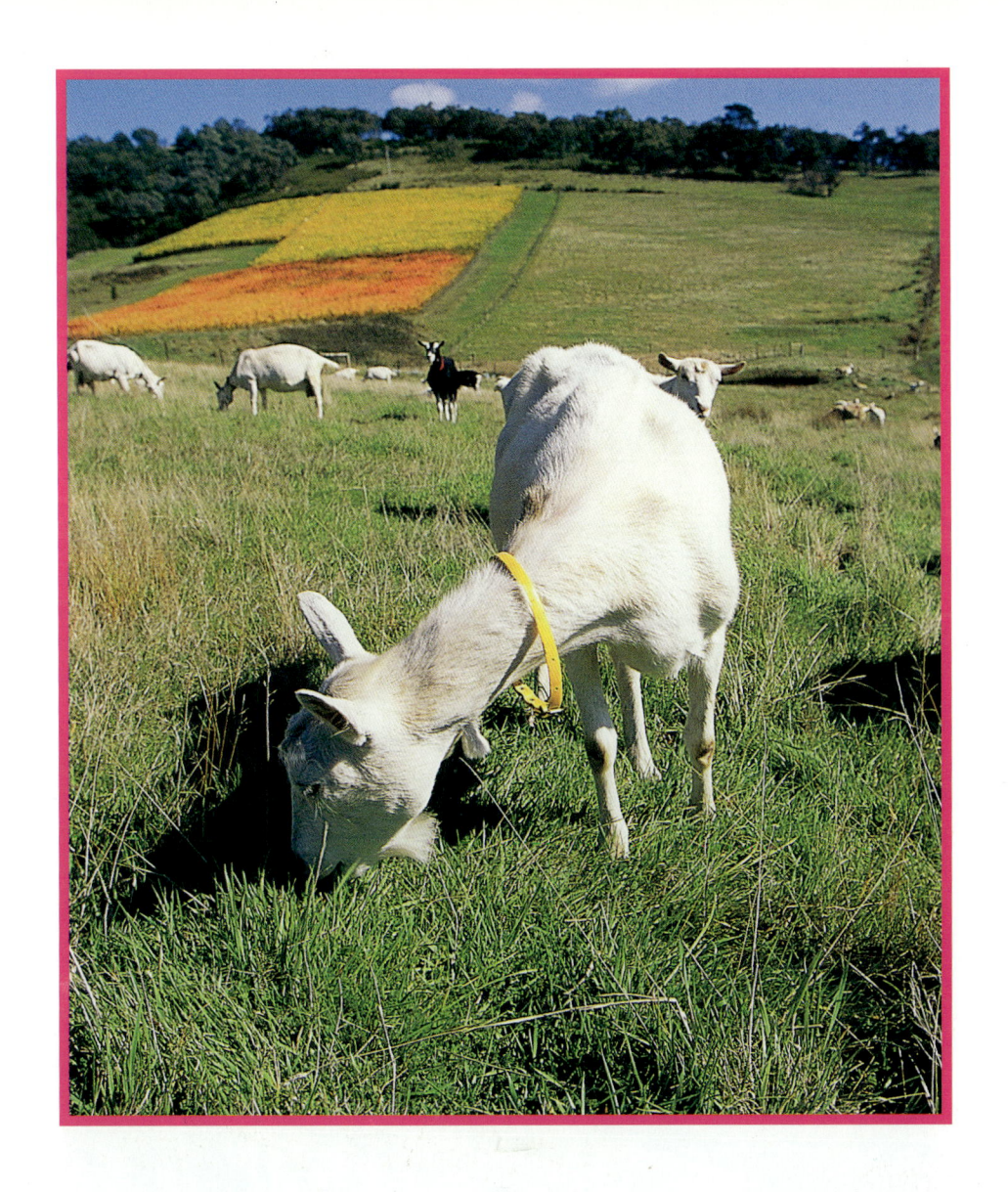

Some people drink milk that comes from goats. Goat milk is also used to make some cheeses and yogurt.

Processing Milk

Workers at a **processing plant** treat cow milk before we drink it. Workers heat milk to 161 degrees Fahrenheit (72 degrees Celsius) for 15 seconds. This pasteurizing process kills **bacteria**.

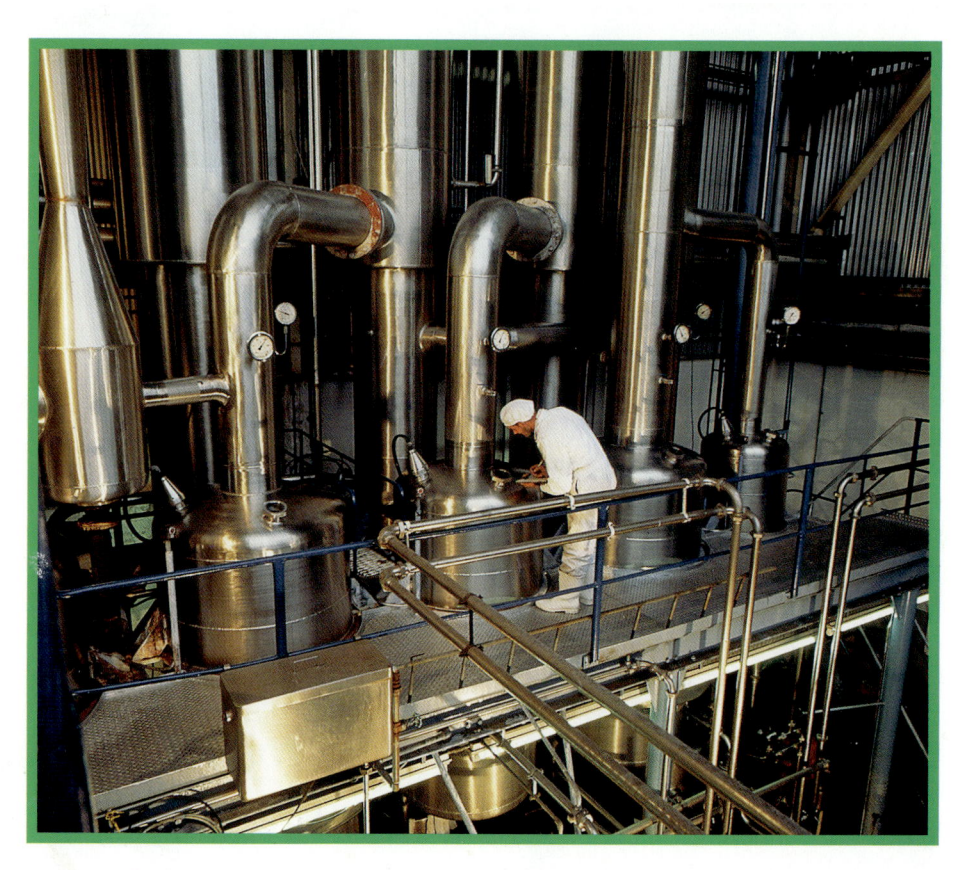

Workers carefully check the temperature when pasteurizing milk.

Milk is stirred in large containers called vats.

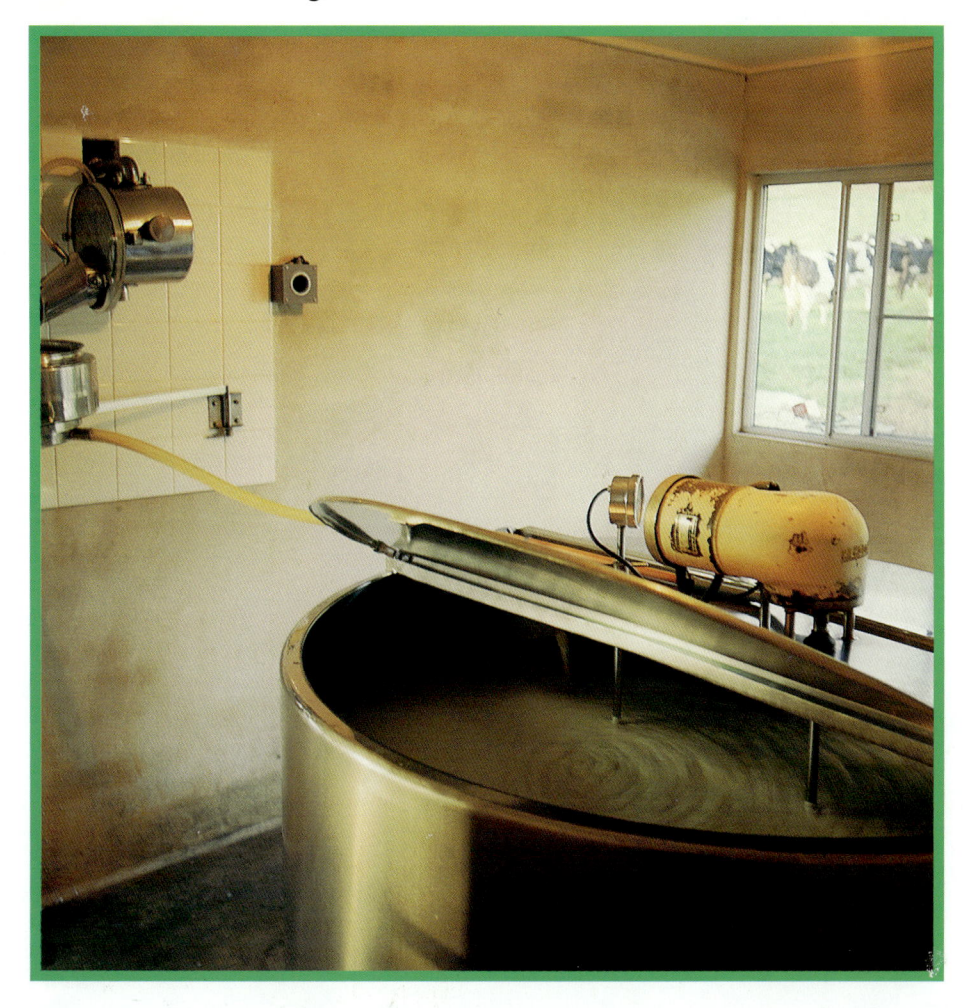

Workers often blend the milk to mix in the milk's fat particles. This process is called homogenizing. Homogenizing makes milk taste rich and smooth.

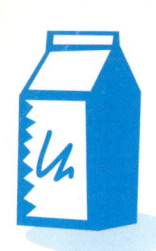

Reduced Fat Milk

Workers make reduced fat milk by letting the milk settle. The fat, or cream, floats to the top. Machines remove the cream.

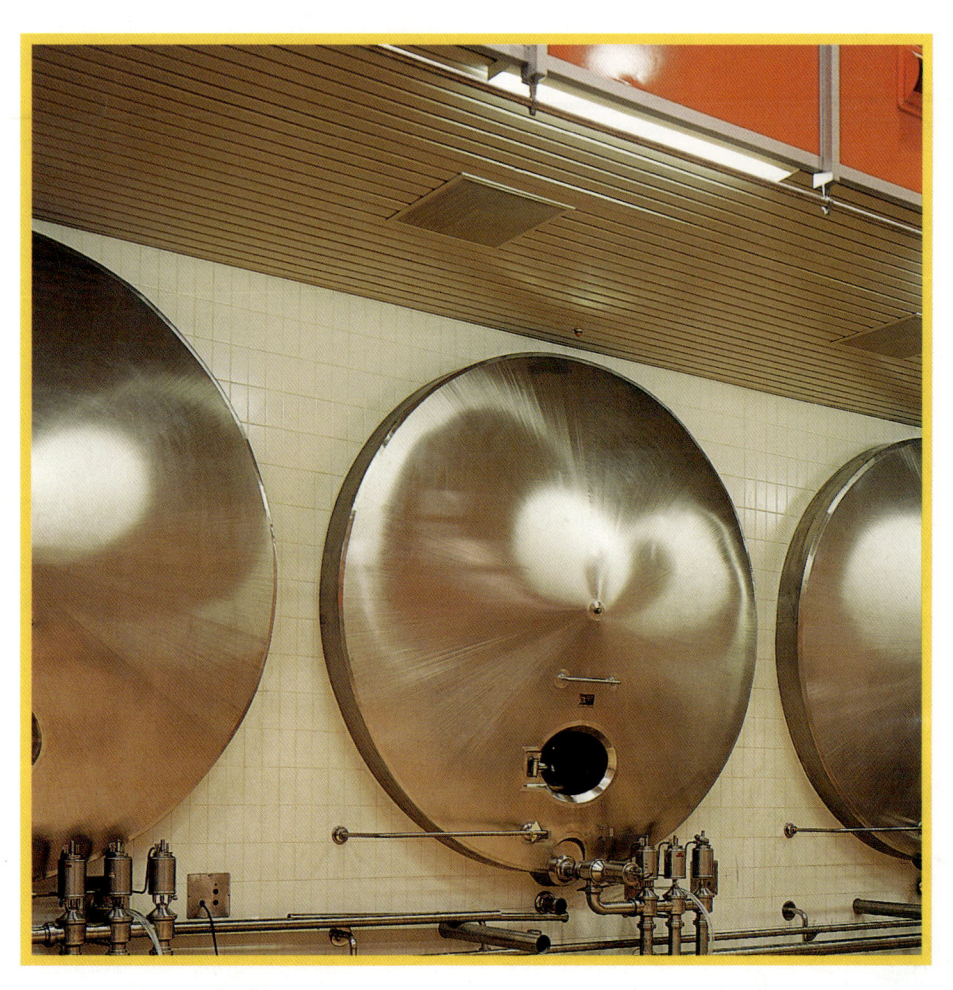

Milk is left to settle in these large vats.

Powdered milk is mixed with water in order to drink.

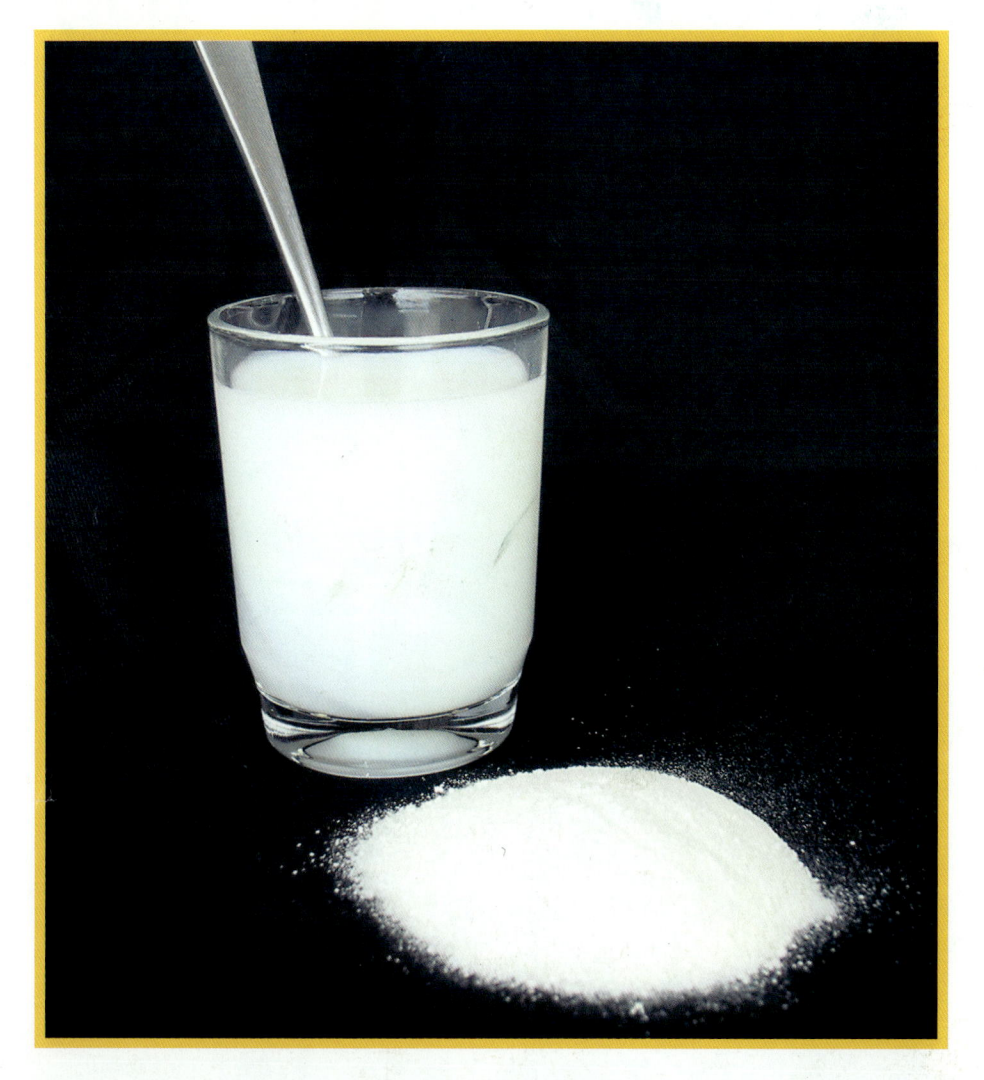

Workers may spin the milk in special machines to remove more fat. Milk can also be dried and made into powder.

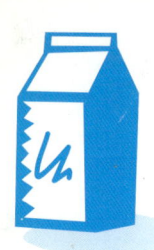

From the Farm to the Factory

Farmers raise large herds of dairy cows on farms. They use machines to milk the cows. The milk is stored and cooled in a large tank.

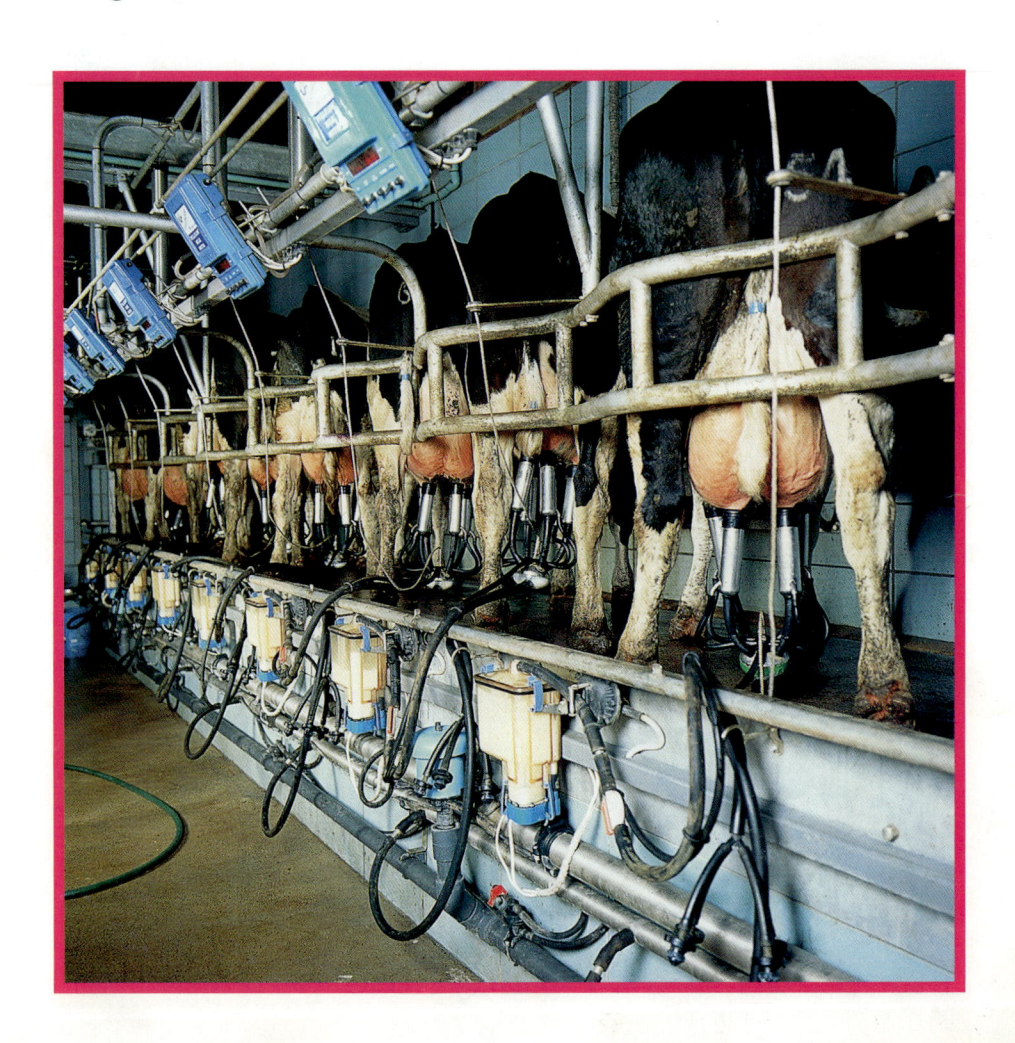

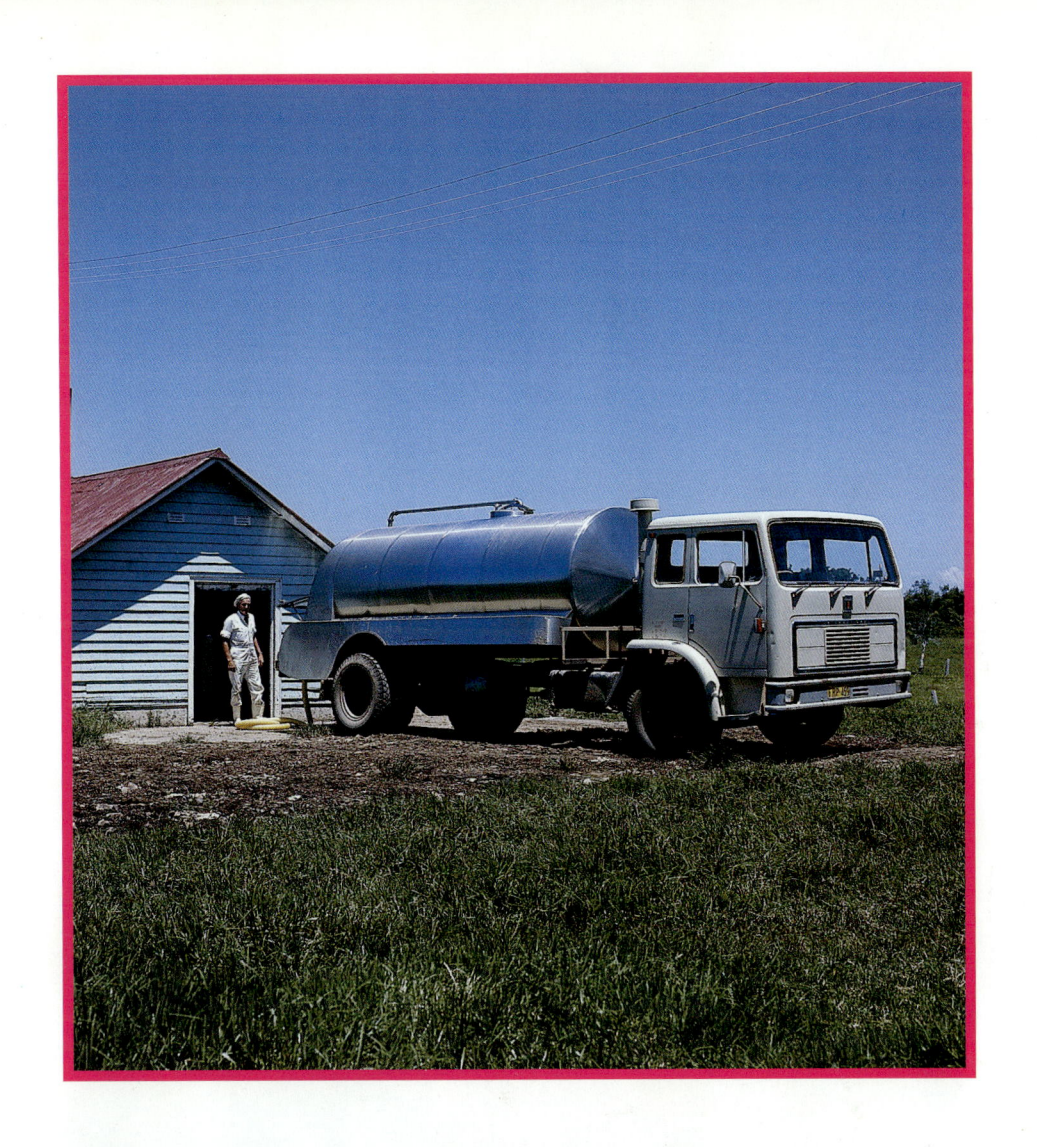

Milk trucks carry milk from farms to a processing plant. At the plant, some milk is bottled. The rest is made into yogurt, cheese, and other foods.

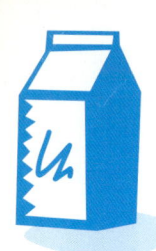

Yogurt

To make yogurt, workers add a bacteria to milk. The mixture becomes thick. Workers often add sugar, fruit, or flavoring to make the yogurt sweet.

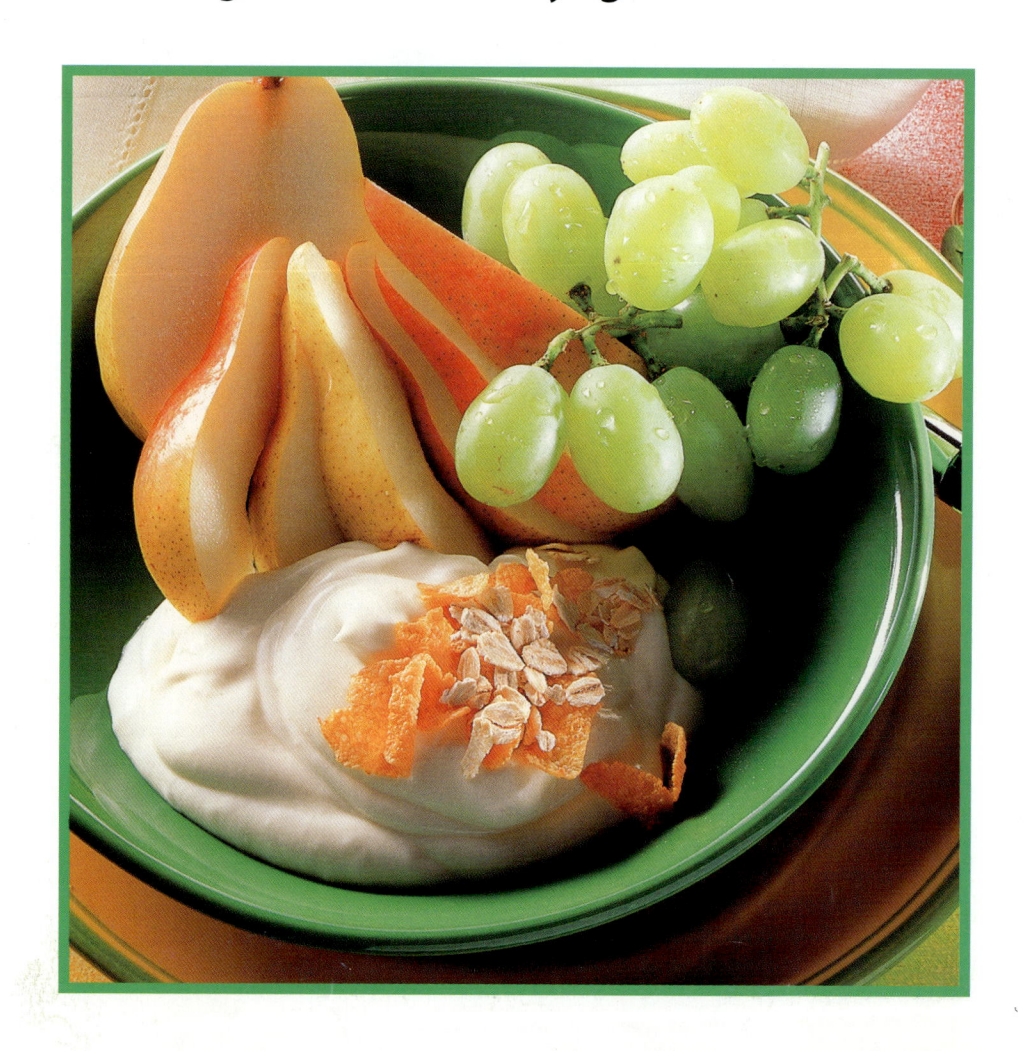

Cheese

Workers make cheese by adding **ingredients** that make the milk separate. The solid parts are curds. The liquid is whey. Workers gather the curds and mold them into blocks of cheese.

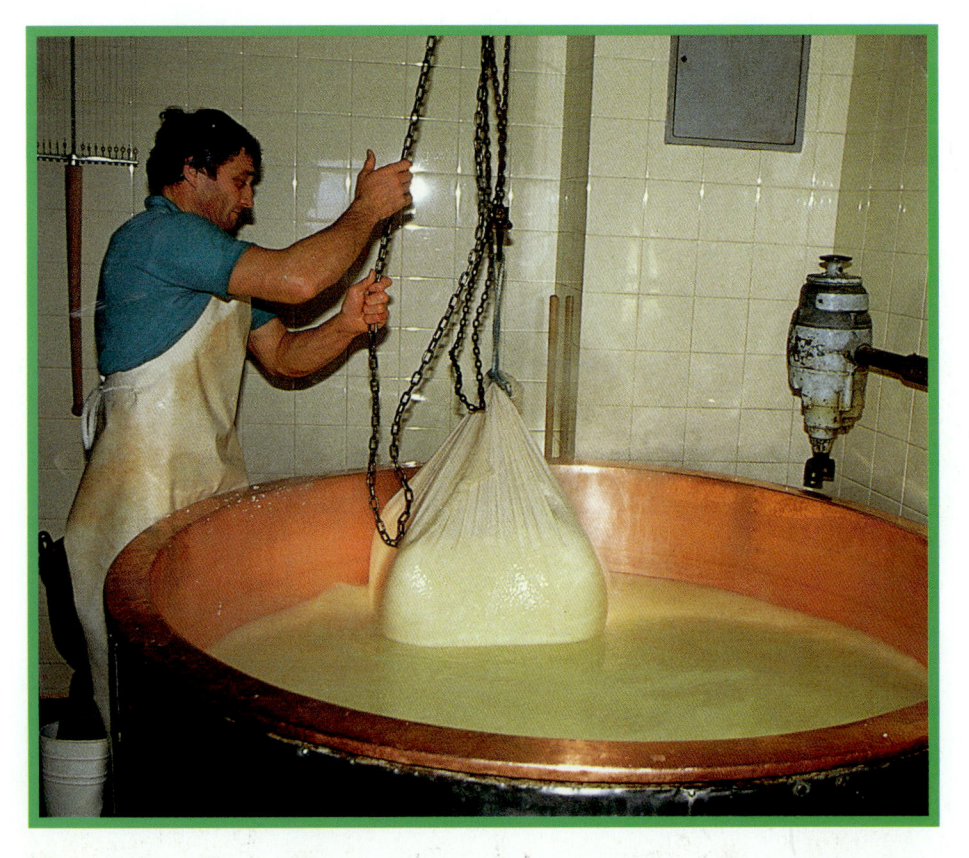

This cheese maker is removing the curds from the whey.

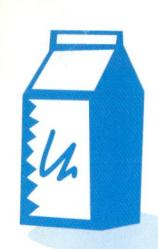

Butter

Workers make butter out of the cream that has been removed from milk. Machines shake or churn the cream until it thickens.

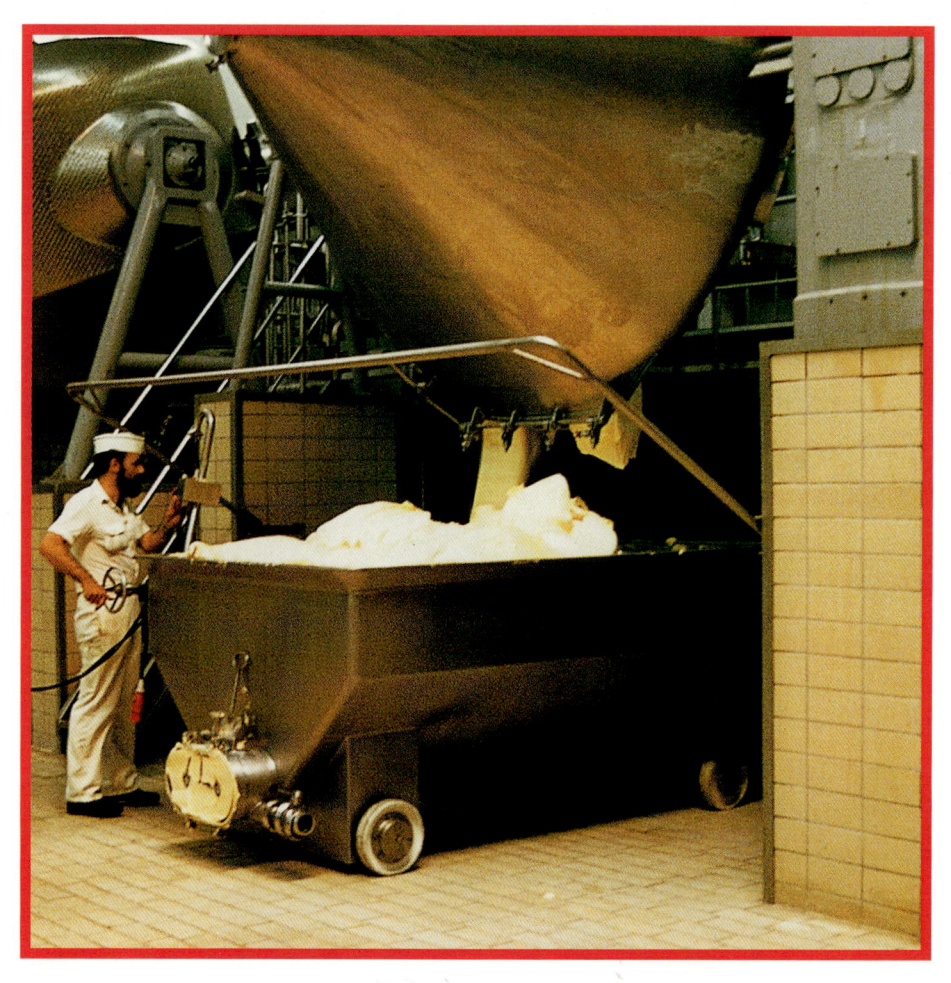

This stainless-steel churn turns cream into butter.

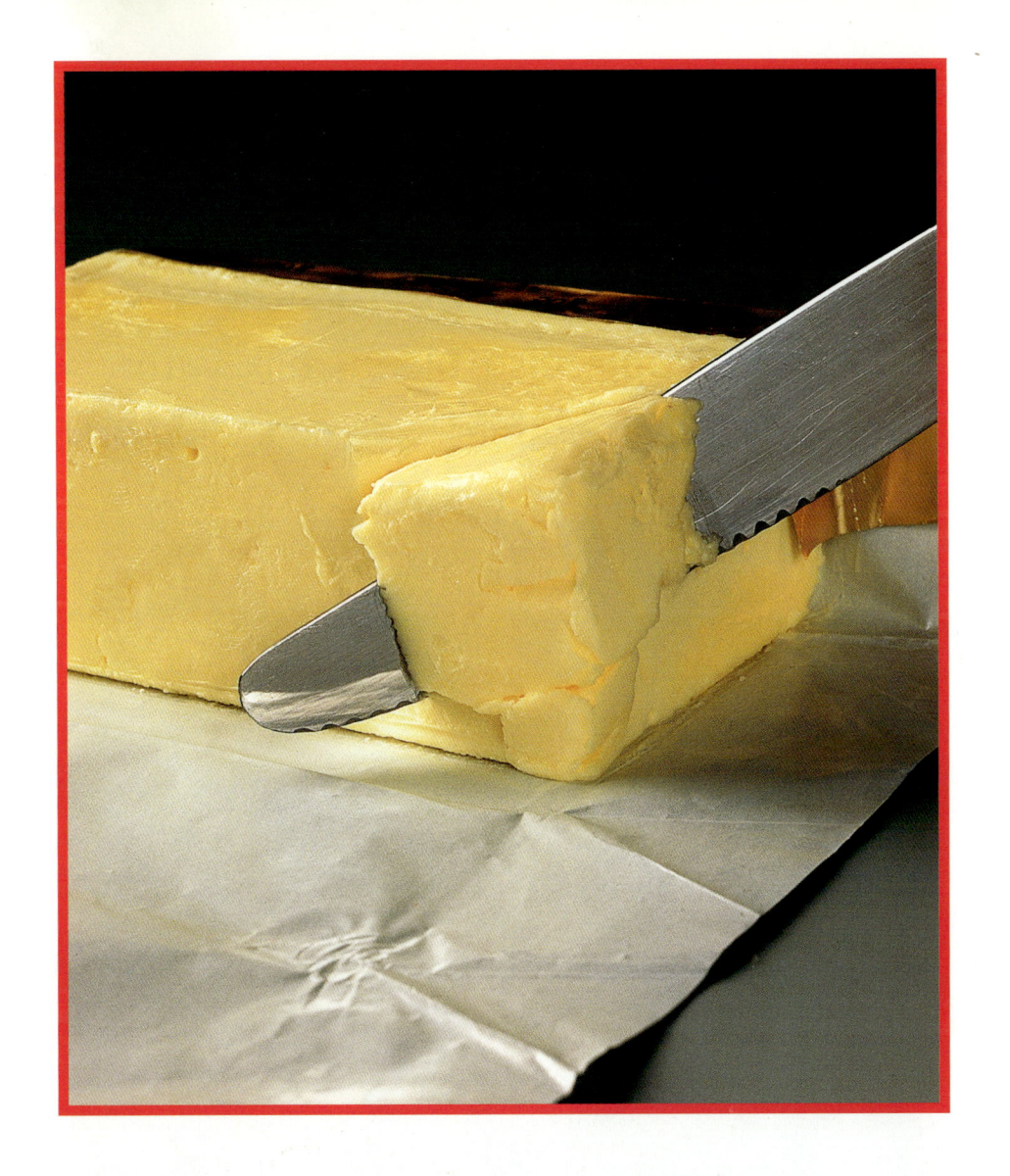

The cream continues to thicken and turns into yellow butter. The liquid left after the butter is removed is called buttermilk.

Drinking and Cooking with Milk

People usually drink plain milk. Sometimes they mix milk with flavors such as chocolate. People also blend milk with fruit to make smoothies.

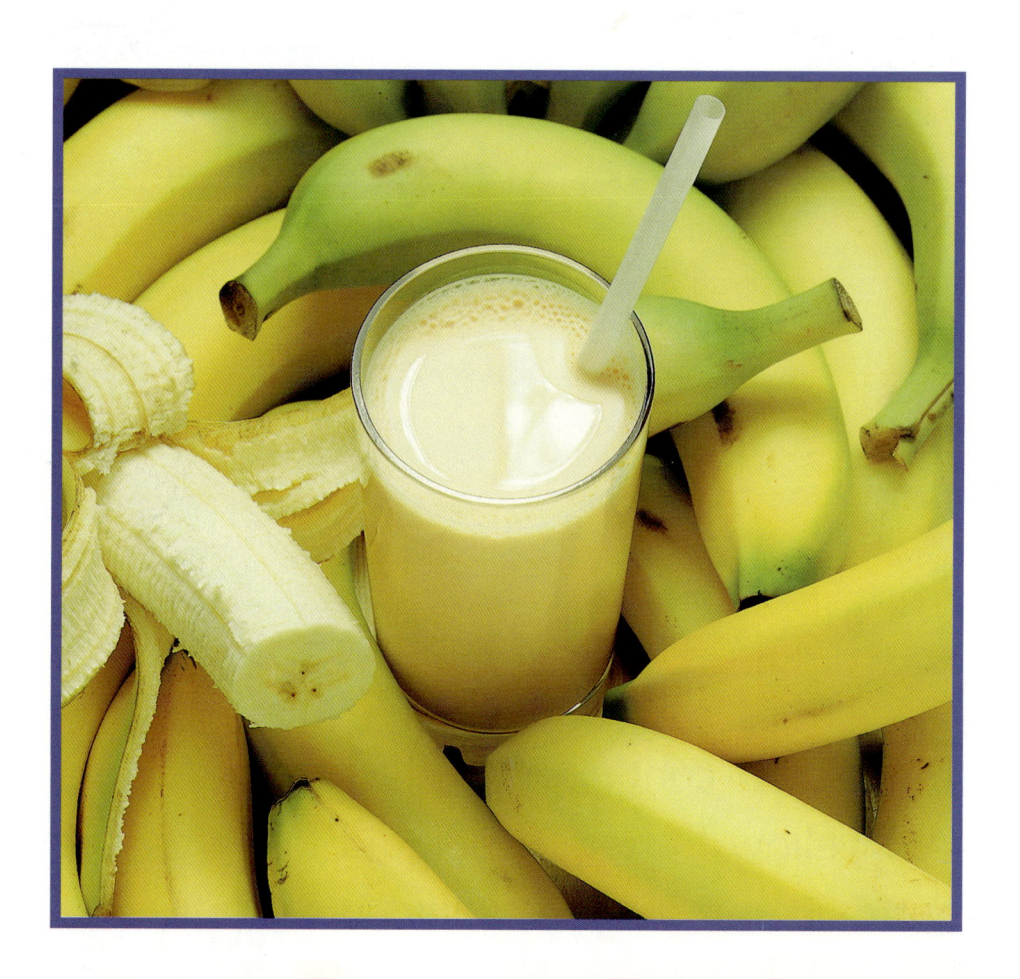

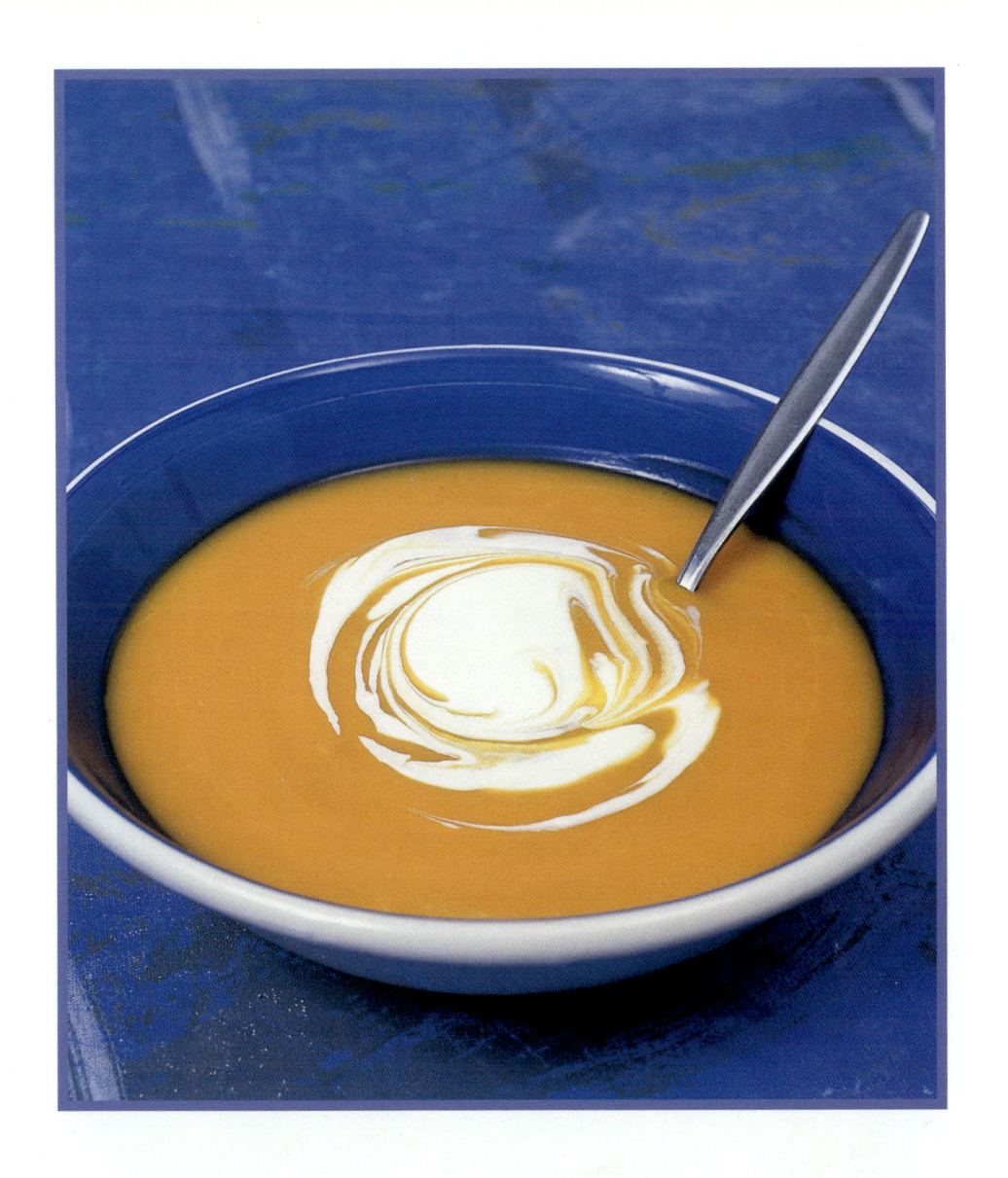

Some soups and sauces contain milk. Milk is used to make custards, puddings, and other foods.

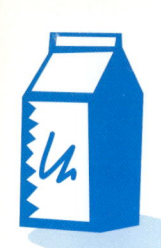

Eating and Cooking with Cheese

Many kinds of cheese are used in cooking. Most pizzas have mozzarella cheese. Feta cheese is often used in Greek cooking. It is made from goat's milk.

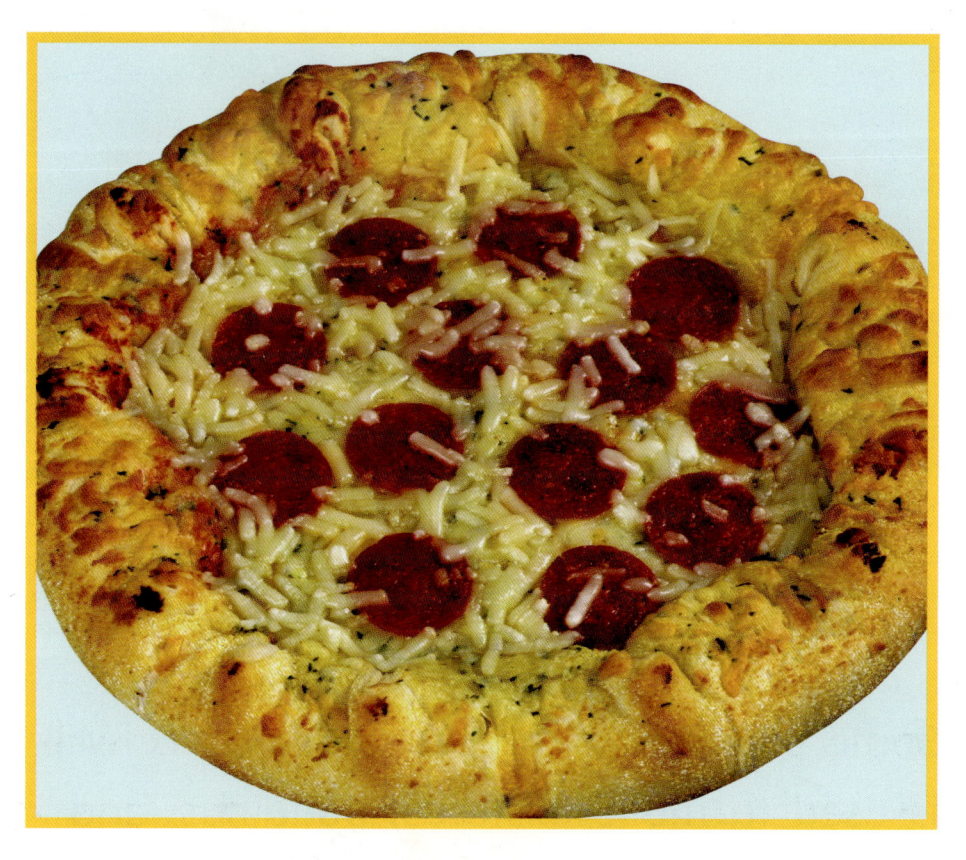

Pizzas are topped with mozzarella cheese.

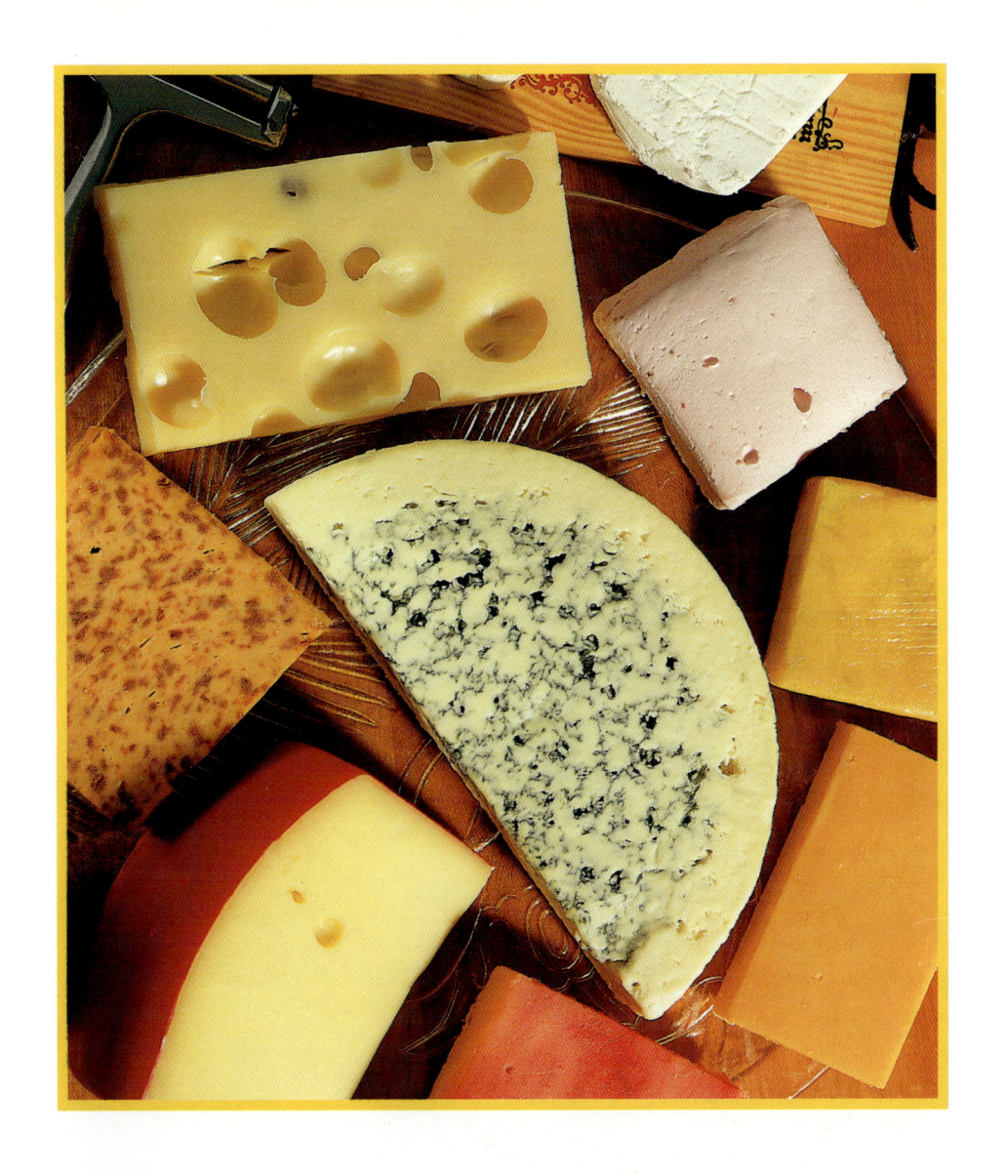

The French are famous for making brie and camembert, two soft cheeses. Swiss cheese is easy to recognize because it has holes.

Cooking with Cream

Cooks often use cream to give foods a rich flavor. They make sauces and soups with cream. People often top their baked potatoes with sour cream.

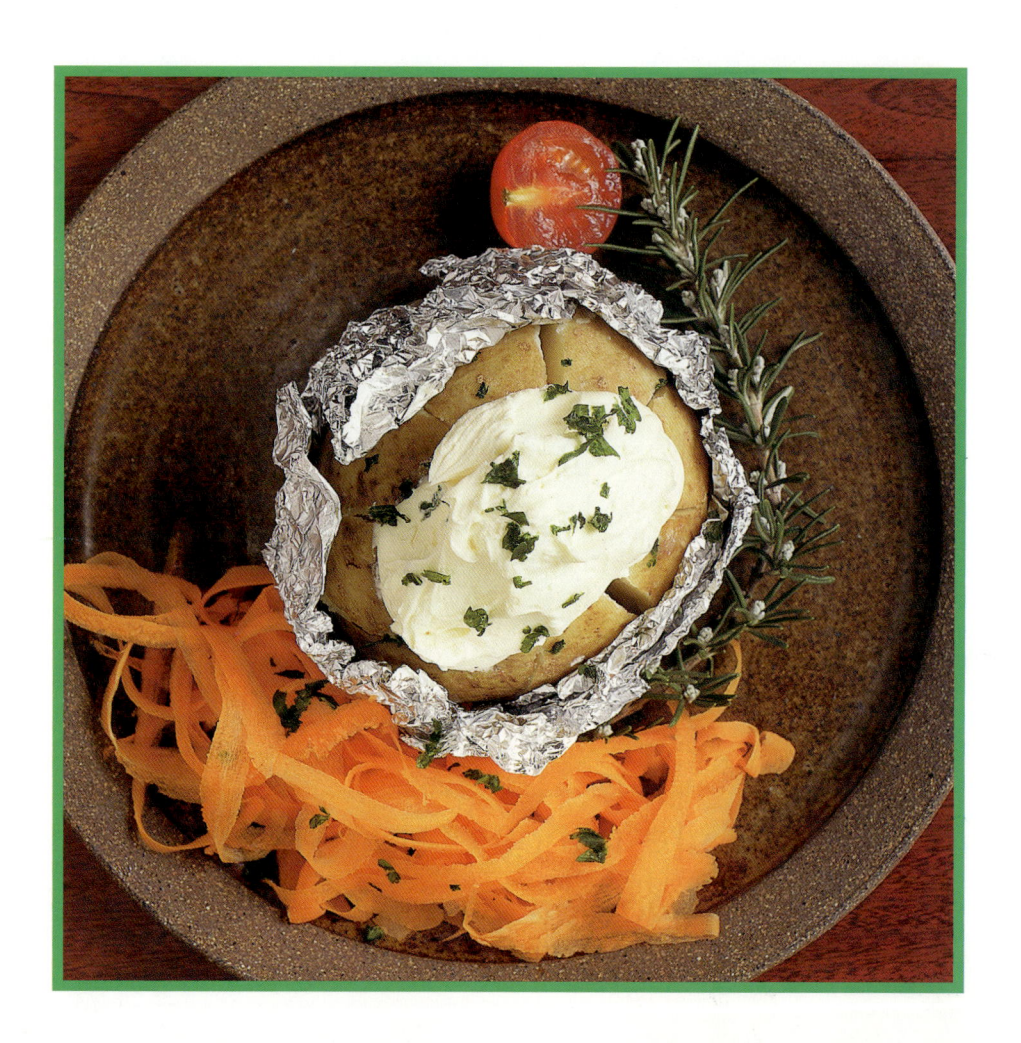

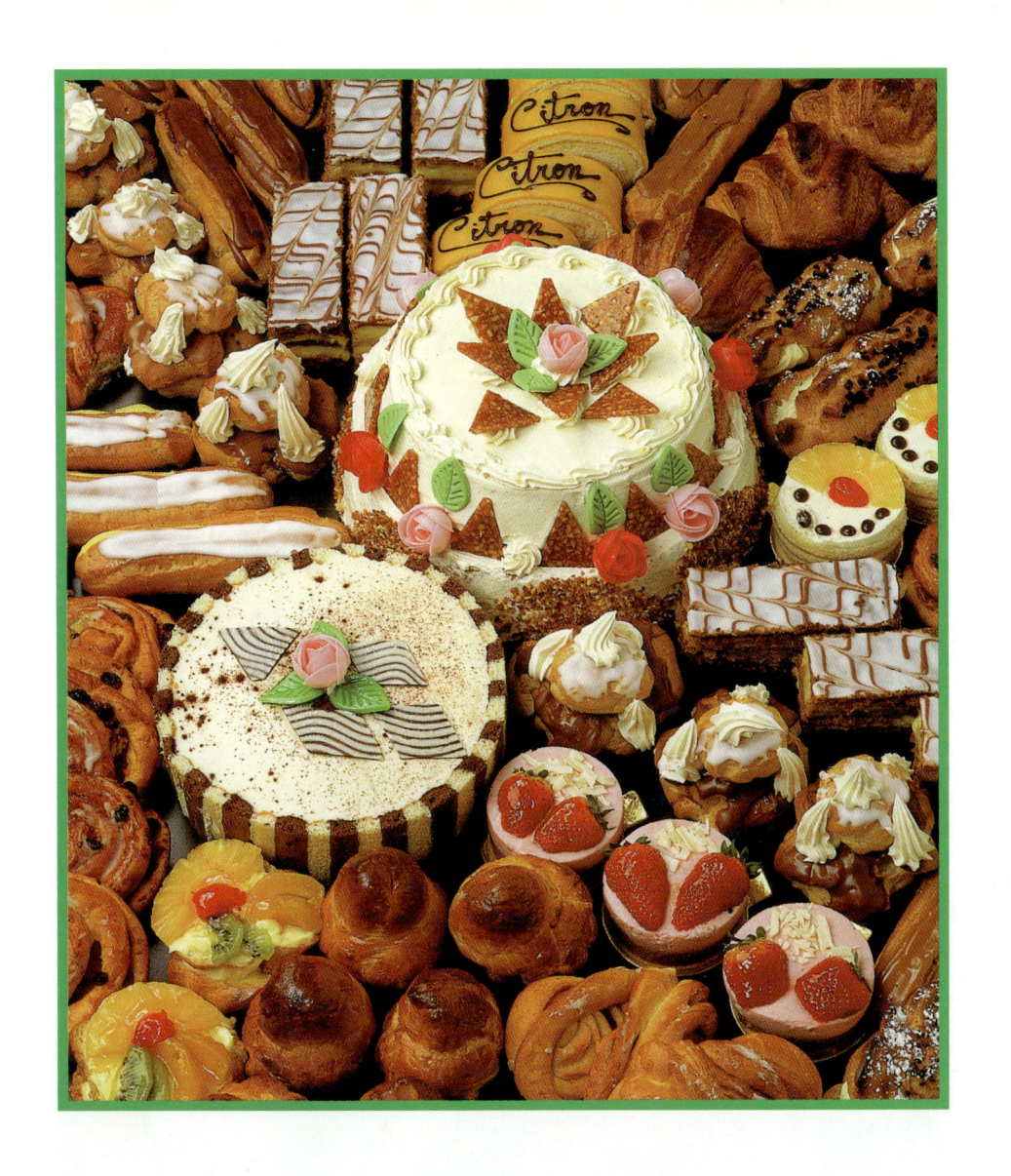

Cream is often used in desserts. It can be whipped into a topping or stirred into frosting.

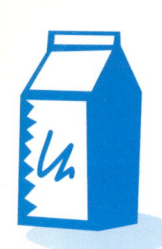

Vegans

Some people do not eat or drink any animal products, including milk. They are called vegans.

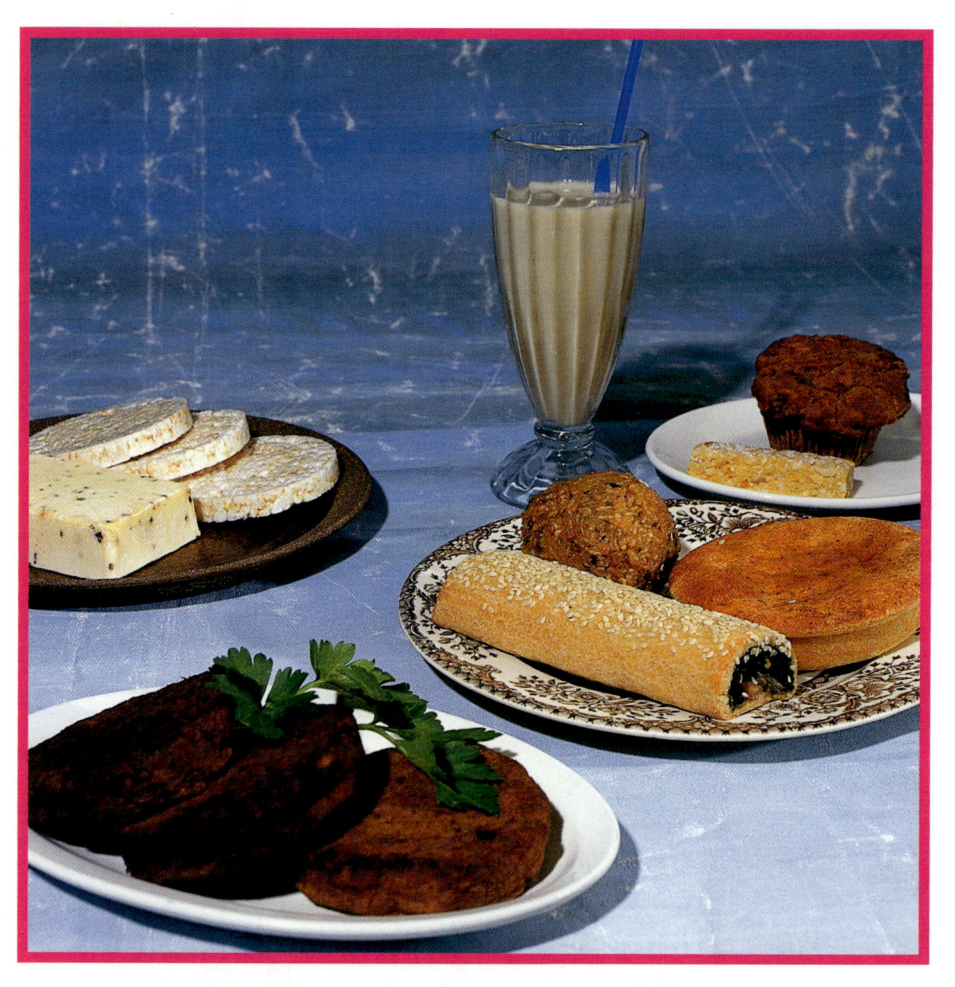

These foods do not contain any animal products.

Some cheeses are made from soybeans.

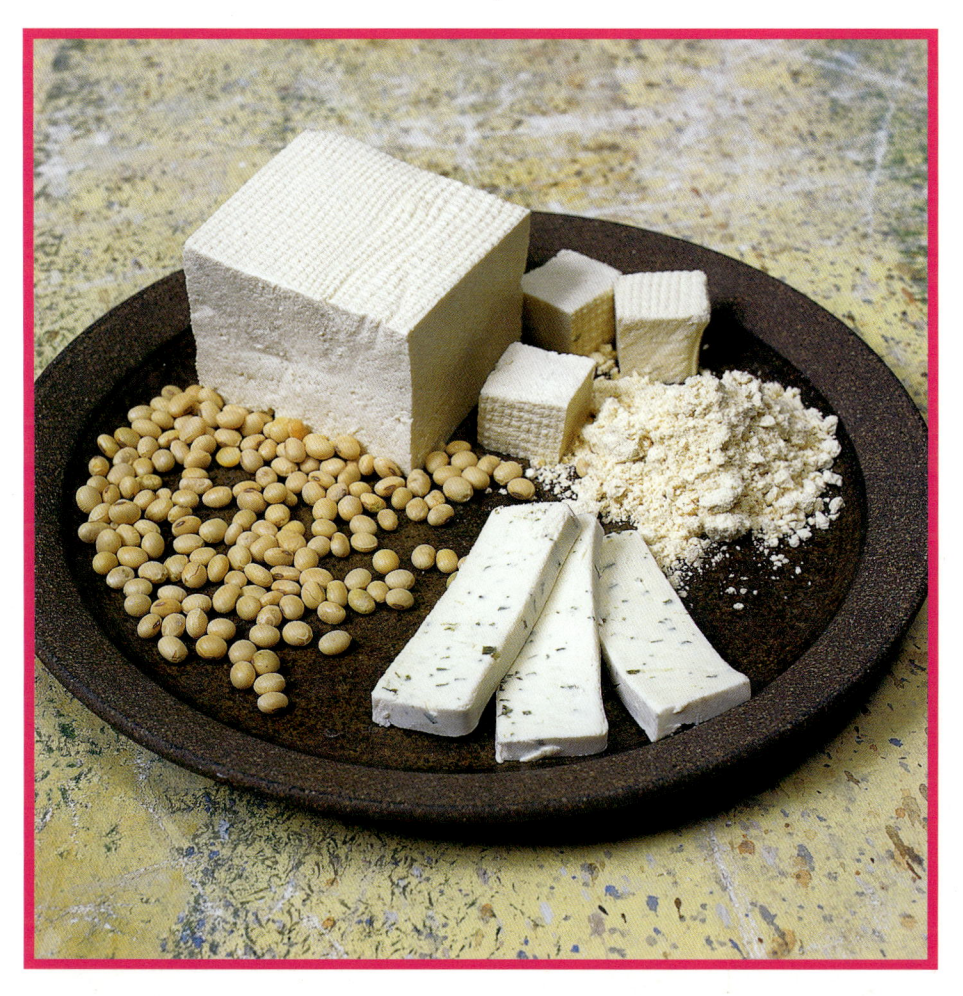

Vegans drink and eat dairy **substitutes**. Soy milk provides the calcium and protein they need to stay healthy. Soy milk and soy cheese are made from soybeans.

The Dairy Group

We should eat two to three servings of dairy products each day.

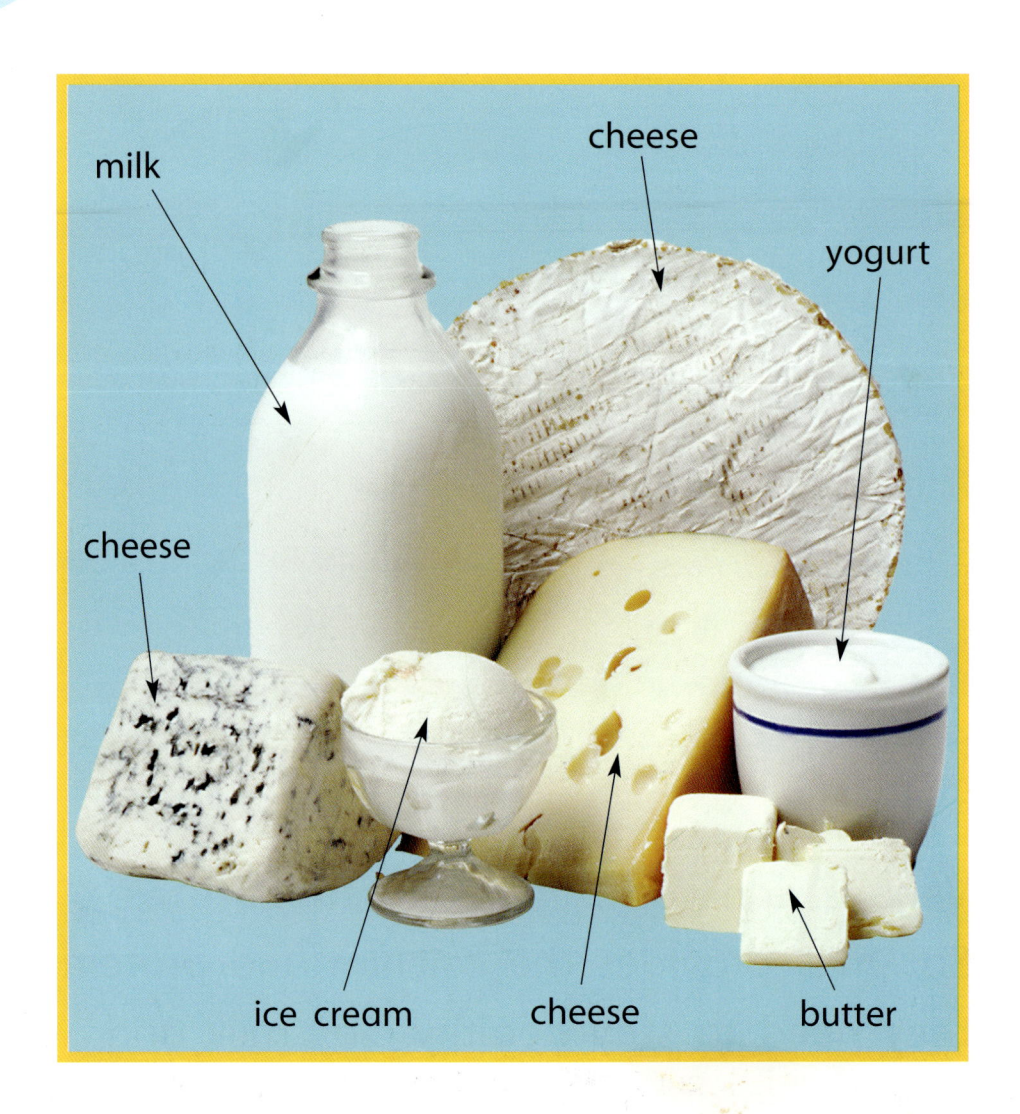

- milk
- cheese
- cheese
- yogurt
- ice cream
- cheese
- butter

Glossary

bacteria a group of very tiny cells that can live all around and inside people, animals, and plants; some types of bacteria are useful, but some cause disease.

carbohydrate an element found in certain foods that gives us energy when eaten; bananas, corn, potatoes, rice, and bread are high in carbohydrates.

ingredient one food that can be combined with others to make something else; recipes use many ingredients.

mineral an element from earth that is found in certain foods; iron and calcium are minerals; we need small amounts of some minerals to stay healthy.

nutrient an element in food that living things need to stay healthy; proteins, minerals, and vitamins are nutrients.

processing plant a factory where products are made in many steps

protein an element found in certain foods that gives us energy when eaten; eggs, meat, cheese, and milk are high in protein.

substitute something used in place of another thing; vegans drink and eat foods made from soy instead of foods made from milk.

vitamin an element found in certain foods; Vitamin C is found in oranges and other foods; we need to eat foods with vitamins to stay healthy.

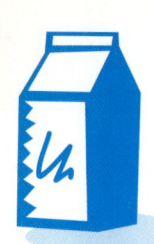

Index

bacteria, 12, 18

butter, 8, 20–21

calcium, 9, 29

carbohydrates, 6

cheese, 8, 11, 17, 19, 24–25, 29

cows, 10, 12, 16

cream, 8, 14, 20–21, 26–27

dairy group, 8, 30

farms, 16–17

food groups, 6–7, 8

food guide pyramid, 7

goats, 11

health, 4–5, 6–7, 9, 29, 30

homogenizing, 13

milk, 8, 10–17, 18, 19, 22–23, 28–29

milk trucks, 17

minerals, 6, 9

nutrients, 6

pasteurizing, 12

powdered milk, 15

processing plant, 12–13, 14–15, 17

proteins, 6, 9, 29

reduced fat milk, 14–15

servings, 30

soy, 29

vegans, 28–29

vitamins, 6, 9

yogurt, 8, 11, 17, 18

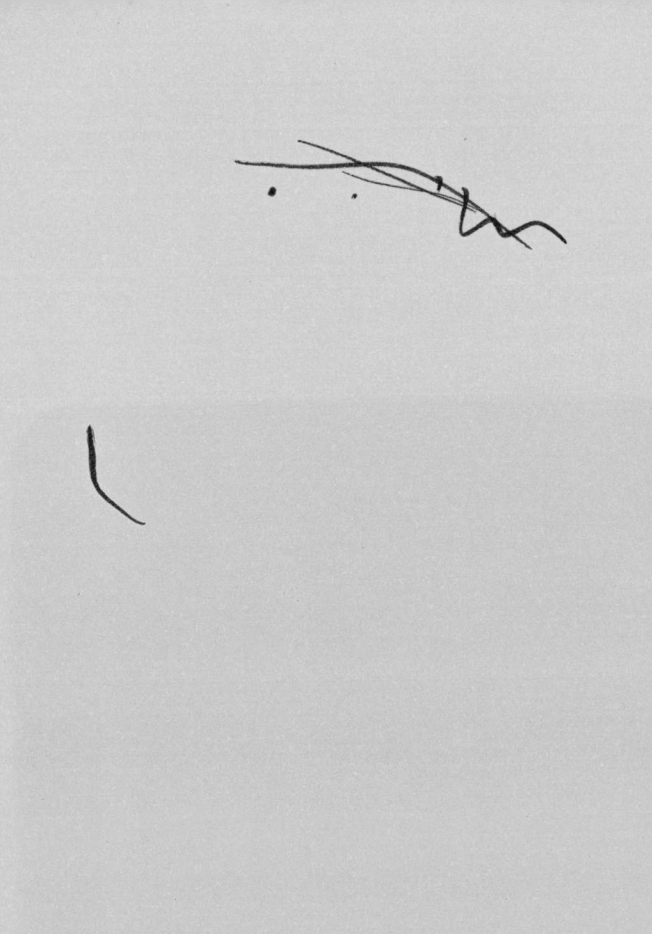